The Diabetic Cookbook

Easy Recipes for a Healthy and Carefree Life
with Delicious Food Low Fat, Low Sugar, And Low Carb

Sophie Kruis

© Copyright 2021 By Sophie Kruis - All rights reserved.

The content contained within this book may not be reproduced, duplicated or transmitted without direct written permission from the author or the publisher.

Under no circumstances will any blame or legal responsibility be held against the publisher, or author, for any damages, reparation, or monetary loss due to the information contained within this book. Either directly or indirectly.

Legal Notice:

This book is copyright protected. This book is only for personal use. You cannot amend, distribute, sell, use, quote or paraphrase any part, or the content within this book, without the consent of the author or publisher.

Disclaimer Notice:

Please note the information contained within this document is for educational and entertainment purposes only. All effort has been executed to present accurate, up to date, and reliable, complete information. No warranties of any kind are declared or implied. Readers acknowledge that the author is not engaging in the rendering of legal, financial, medical or professional advice. The content within this book has been derived from various sources. Please consult a licensed professional before attempting any techniques outlined in this book.

By reading this document, the reader agrees that under no circumstances is the author responsible for any losses, direct or indirect, which are incurred as a result of the use of information contained within this document, including, but not limited to, errors, omissions, or inaccuracies.

Table Of Contents

INTRODUCTION 6

BREAKFAST RECIPES 9
1. Salty Macadamia Chocolate Smoothie 9
2. Basil and Tomato Baked Eggs 11
3. Cinnamon and Coconut Porridge 13
4. An Omelet of Swiss chard 15

APPETIZER RECIPES 18
5. Parmesan Broiled Flounder 18
6. Fish with Fresh Tomato - Basil Sauce 20
7. Baked Chicken 22
8. Seared Chicken with Roasted Vegetables 24
9. Fish Simmered in Tomato-Pepper Sauce 26
10. Cheese Potato and Pea Casserole 28
11. Oven-Fried Tilapia 30
12. Chicken with Coconut Sauce 32

FIRST COURSE RECIPES 35
13. Chicken and Cornmeal Dumplings 35
14. Chicken and Pepperoni 38
15. Chicken and Sausage Gumbo 40
16. Chicken, Barley, and Leek Stew 42

SECOND COURSE RECIPES 45
17. Sweet and Sour Onions 45
18. Sautéed Apples and Onions 47
19. Zucchini Noodles with Portabella Mushrooms 49
20. Grilled Tempeh with Pineapple 51
21. Courgettes In Cider Sauce 53
22. Baked Mixed Mushrooms 55

SIDE DISH RECIPES 59
23. Parsley Tabbouleh 59
24. Garlic Sautéed Spinach 61
25. French Lentils 63
26. Grain-Free Berry Cobbler 65
27. Coffee-Steamed Carrots 67

28.	Rosemary Potatoes	68
29.	Corn on the Cob	70

SOUPS & STEWS 73

30.	Alkaline Pumpkin Tomato Soup	73
31.	Alkaline Pumpkin Coconut Soup	75
32.	Cold Cauliflower-Coconut Soup	77
33.	Raw Avocado-Broccoli Soup with Cashew Nuts	79
34.	White Bean Soup	81

DESSERTS 84

35.	Pumpkin & Banana Ice Cream	84
36.	Brulee Oranges	85
37.	Frozen Lemon & Blueberry	87
38.	Peanut Butter Choco Chip Cookies	88
39.	Watermelon Sherbet	90
40.	Strawberry & Mango Ice Cream	91
41.	Sparkling Fruit Drink	92
42.	Detox Berry Smoothie	93

OTHER DIABETIC RECIPES 96

43.	Bruschetta	96
44.	Cream Buns with Strawberries	98
45.	Blueberry Buns	100
46.	Cauliflower Potato Mash	102
47.	French toast in Sticks	104
48.	Muffins Sandwich	106
49.	Bacon BBQ	108

CONCLUSION 110

Introduction

People with diabetes often think they need to become strictly focused on avoiding sugar or carbohydrates and neglect to consider the nutritional quality of their diet.

While it's true that carbohydrates have the greatest impact on blood sugar, it is the diet as a whole that contributes to health, weight management, and blood sugar control. Strictly limiting carbohydrates found in fruit and whole grains while eating a diet high in saturated fat and sodium will not promote optimal health.

Diabetes is a condition where the body is no longer able to self-regulate blood glucose. When you eat a food that contains carbohydrates, whether it comes from honey, an apple, or brown rice, the body breaks it down into sugar (also called glucose) during digestion. This glucose passes through the walls of the intestines into the blood, which causes blood sugar (the amount of glucose circulating in the blood) to rise.

In response, the pancreas secretes a hormone called insulin. The role of insulin is to lower the blood sugar back to normal levels. It does this by moving the sugar out of the blood and into the cells, where it is used for energy. Think of insulin as a key that unlocks the doors to the cells. But if you have diabetes, either the body doesn't make enough insulin, or the cells don't respond to the insulin. This causes the blood sugar to build up in the bloodstream, resulting in high blood sugar.

A diabetes diagnosis means that the pancreas is not able to produce enough insulin to keep up with this resistance—and insulin deficiency is the result. If your body can't make enough insulin, blood sugar levels become elevated. Long-term elevated blood sugar levels can affect almost every system in the body. This is why it is so important to work with your healthcare team to come up with the best treatment plan for you and for you to take the leading part in your plan by eating healthy, staying physically active, and losing weight if necessary.

Breakfast Recipes

1. Salty Macadamia Chocolate Smoothie

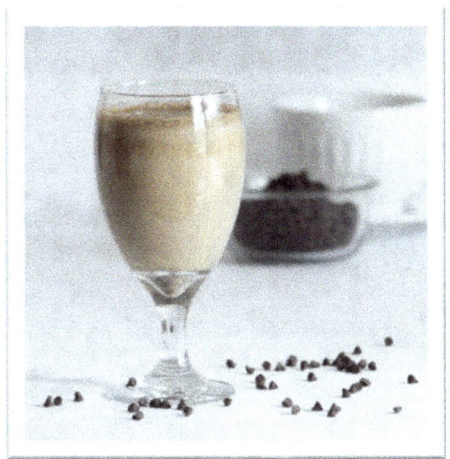

Preparation Time: 5 minutes
Cooking Time: Nil
Servings: 1
Ingredients:
- 2 tablespoons macadamia nuts, salted
- 1/3 cup chocolate whey protein powder, low carb
- 1 cup almond milk, unsweetened

Directions:
1. Add the listed ingredients to your blender and blend until you have a smooth mixture
2. Chill and enjoy it!

Nutrition: Calories: 165; Fat: 2g; Carbohydrates: 1g; Protein: 12g

2. Basil and Tomato Baked Eggs

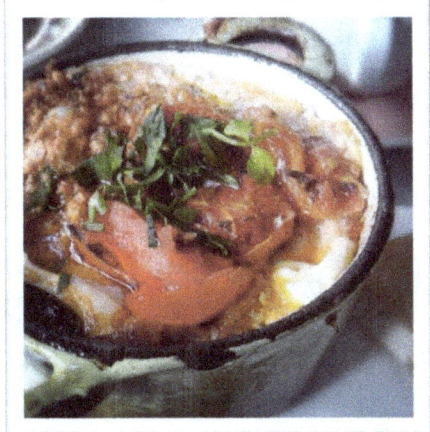

Preparation Time: 10 minutes

Cooking Time: 15 minutes

Servings: 4

Ingredients:
- 1 garlic clove, minced
- 1 cup canned tomatoes
- ¼ cup fresh basil leaves, roughly chopped
- 1/2 teaspoon chili powder
- 1 tablespoon olive oil
- 4 whole eggs
- Salt and pepper to taste

Directions:
1. Preheat your oven to 375 degrees F
2. Take a small baking dish and grease with olive oil
3. Add garlic, basil, tomatoes chili, olive oil into a dish and stir
4. Crackdown eggs into a dish, keeping space between the two
5. Sprinkle the whole dish with salt and pepper
6. Place in oven and cook for 12 minutes until eggs are set and tomatoes are bubbling
7. Serve with basil on top
8. Enjoy!

Nutrition: Calories: 235; Fat: 16g; Carbohydrates: 7g; Protein: 14g

3. Cinnamon and Coconut Porridge

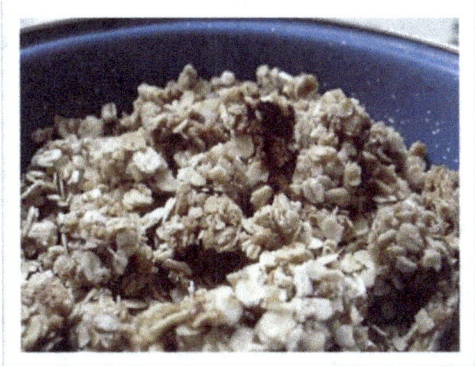

Preparation Time: 5 minutes

Cooking Time: 5 minutes

Servings: 4

Ingredients:

- 2 cups of water
- 1 cup 36% heavy cream
- 1/2 cup unsweetened dried coconut, shredded
- 2 tablespoons flaxseed meal
- 1 tablespoon butter
- 1 and 1/2 teaspoon stevia
- 1 teaspoon cinnamon
- Salt to taste
- Toppings as blueberries

Directions:

1. Add the listed ingredients to a small pot, mix well
2. Transfer pot to stove and place it over medium-low heat
3. Bring to mix to a slow boil
4. Stir well and remove the heat
5. Divide the mix into equal servings and let them sit for 10 minutes
6. Top with your desired toppings and enjoy!

Nutrition: Calories: 171; Fat: 16g; Carbohydrates: 6g; Protein: 2g

4. An Omelet of Swiss chard

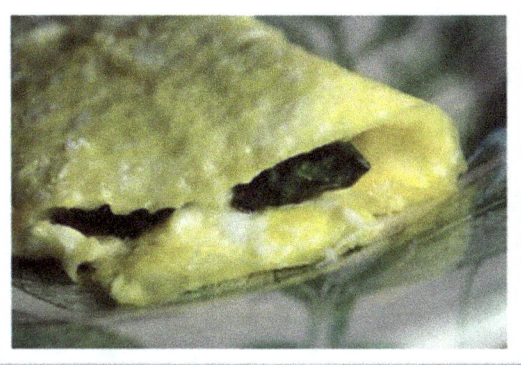

Preparation Time: 5 minutes

Cooking Time: 5 minutes

Servings: 4

Ingredients:

- 4 eggs, lightly beaten
- 4 cups Swiss chard, sliced
- 2 tablespoons butter
- 1/2 teaspoon garlic salt
- Fresh pepper

Directions:

1. Take a non-stick frying pan and place it over medium-low heat
2. Once the butter melts, add Swiss chard and stir cook for 2 minutes

3. Pour egg into the pan and gently stir them into Swiss chard
4. Season with garlic salt and pepper
5. Cook for 2 minutes
6. Serve and enjoy!

Nutrition: Calories: 260; Fat: 21g; Carbohydrates: 4g; Protein: 14g

Appetizer Recipes

5. Parmesan Broiled Flounder

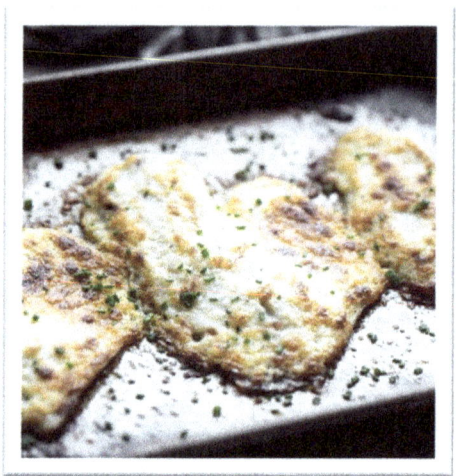

Preparation Time: 10 minutes

Cooking Time: 7 minutes

Serving: 2

Ingredients:

- 2 (4-oz) flounder

- 1,5 tbsp Parmesan cheese

- 1,5 tbsp mayonnaise

- 1/8 tsp soy sauce

- 1/4 tsp chili sauce

- 1/8 tsp salt-free lemon-pepper seasoning

Directions:

1. Preheat flounder.
2. Mix cheese, reduced-fat mayonnaise, soy sauce, chili sauce, seasoning.
3. Put fish on a baking sheet coated with cooking spray, sprinkle with salt and pepper.
4. Spread Parmesan mixture over flounder.
5. Broil 6 to 8 minutes or until a crust appears on the fish.

Nutrition: 200 Calories; 17g Fat; 7g Carbohydrate

6. Fish with Fresh Tomato - Basil Sauce

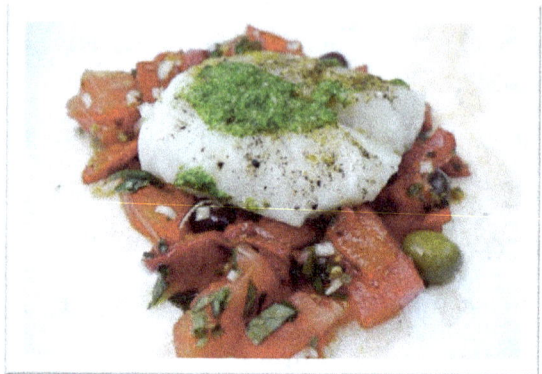

Preparation Time: 10 minutes

Cooking Time: 15 minutes

Serving: 2

Ingredients:

- 2 (4-oz) tilapia fillets
- 1 tbsp fresh basil, chopped
- 1/8 tsp salt
- 1 pinch of crushed red pepper
- 1 cup cherry tomatoes, chopped
- 2 tsp extra virgin olive oil

Directions:

1. Preheat oven to 400°F.
2. Arrange rinsed and patted dry fish fillets on foil (coat a foil baking sheet with cooking spray).

3. Sprinkle tilapia fillets with salt and red pepper.
4. Bake 12 - 15 minutes.
5. Meanwhile, mix leftover ingredients in a saucepan.
6. Cook over medium-high heat until tomatoes are tender.
7. Top fish fillets properly with tomato mixture.

Nutrition: 130 Calories; 30g Protein; 1g Carbohydrates

7. Baked Chicken

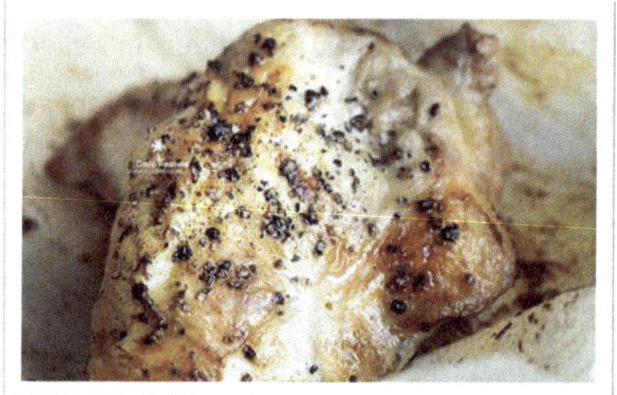

Preparation Time: 15 minutes

Cooking Time: 25 minutes

Serving: 4

Ingredients:

- 2 (6-oz) bone-in chicken breasts
- 1/8 tsp salt
- 1/8 tsp pepper
- 3 tsp extra virgin olive oil
- 1/2 tsp dried oregano
- 7 pitted kalamata olives
- 1 cup cherry tomatoes
- 1/2 cup onion
- 1 (9-oz) pkg frozen artichoke hearts

- 1 lemon

Directions:

1. Preheat oven to 400°F.
2. Sprinkle chicken with pepper, salt, and oregano.
3. Heat oil, add chicken and cook until it browned.
4. Place chicken in a baking dish. Arrange tomatoes, coarsely chopped olives, and onion, artichokes and lemon cut into wedges around the chicken.
5. Bake 20 minutes or until chicken is done and vegetables are tender.

Nutrition: 160 Calories; 3g Fat; 1g Carbohydrates

8. Seared Chicken with Roasted Vegetables

Preparation Time: 20 minutes

Cooking Time: 30 minutes

Serving: 1

Ingredients:

- 1 (8-oz) boneless, skinless chicken breasts
- 3/4 lb. small Brussels sprouts
- 2 large carrots
- 1 large red bell pepper
- 1 small red onion
- 2 cloves garlic halved
- 2 tbsp extra virgin olive oil
- 1/2 tsp dried dill
- 1/4 tsp pepper
- 1/4 tsp salt

Directions:

1. Preheat oven to 425°F.
2. Match Brussels sprouts cut in half, red onion cut into wedges, sliced carrots, bell pepper cut into pieces and halved garlic on a baking sheet.
3. Sprinkle with 1 tbsp oil and with 1/8 tsp salt and 1/8 tsp pepper. Bake until well-roasted, cool slightly.

4. In the Meantime, sprinkle chicken with dill, remaining 1/8 tsp salt and 1/8 tsp pepper. Cook until chicken is done. Put roasted vegetables with drippings over chicken.

Nutrition:170 Calories; 7g Fat; 12g Protein

9. Fish Simmered in Tomato-Pepper Sauce

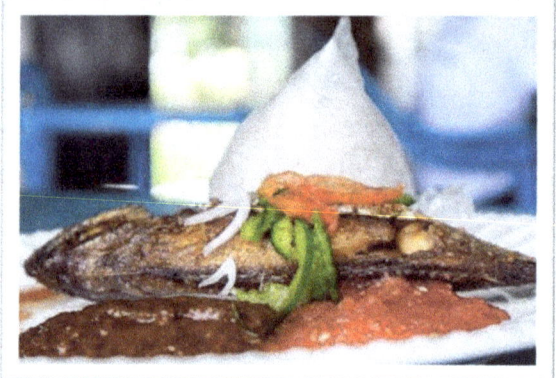

Preparation Time: 5 minutes

Cooking Time: 10 minutes

Serving: 2

Ingredients:

- 2 (4-oz) cod fillets
- 1 big tomato
- 1/3 cup red peppers (roasted)
- 3 tbsp almonds
- 2 cloves garlic
- 2 tbsp fresh basil leaves
- 2 tbsp extra virgin olive oil
- 1/4 tsp salt
- 1/8 tsp pepper

Directions:

1. Toast sliced almonds in a pan until fragrant.
2. Grind almonds, basil, minced garlic, 1-2 tsp oil in a food processor until finely ground.
3. Add coarsely-chopped tomato and red peppers; grind until smooth.
4. Season fish with salt and pepper.
5. Cook in hot oil in a large pan over medium-high heat until fish is browned. Pour sauce around fish. Cook 6 minutes more.

Nutrition: 90 Calories; 5g Fat; 7g Carbohydrates

10. Cheese Potato and Pea Casserole

Preparation Time: 10 minutes

Cooking Time: 35 minutes

Serving: 3

Ingredients:

- 1 tbsp olive oil
- ¾ lb. red potatoes
- ¾ cup green peas
- ½ cup red onion
- ¼ tsp dried rosemary
- ¼ tsp salt
- 1/8 tsp pepper

Directions:

1. Prepare oven to 350°F.
2. Cook 1 tsp oil in a skillet. Stir in thinly sliced onions and cook. Remove from pan.
3. Situate half of the thinly sliced potatoes and onions in bottom of skillet; top with peas, crushed dried rosemary, and 1/8 tsp each salt and pepper.
4. Place remaining potatoes and onions on top. Season with remaining 1/8 tsp salt.
5. Bake 35 minutes, pour remaining 2 tsp oil and sprinkle with cheese.

Nutrition: 80 Calories; 2g Protein; 18g Carbohydrates

11. Oven-Fried Tilapia

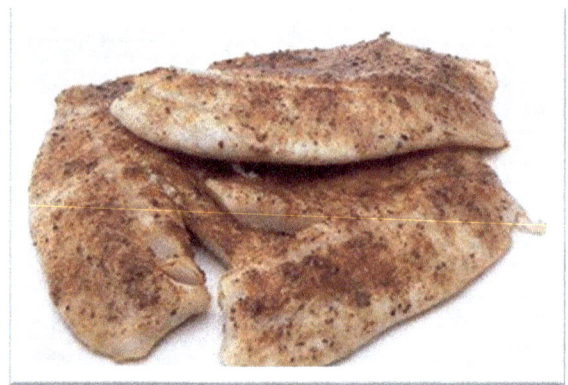

Preparation Time: 7 minutes

Cooking Time: 15 minutes

Serving: 2

Ingredients:

- 2 (4-oz) tilapia fillets
- 1/4 cup yellow cornmeal
- 2 tbsp light ranch dressing
- 1 tbsp canola oil
- 1 tsp dill (dried)
- 1/8 tsp salt

Directions:

1. Preheat oven to 425°F. Brush both sides of rinsed and patted dry tilapia fish fillets with dressing.
2. Combine cornmeal, oil, dill, and salt.

3. Sprinkle fish fillets with cornmeal mixture.
4. Put fish on a prepared baking sheet.
5. Bake 15 minutes.

Nutrition: 96 Calories; 21g Protein; 2g Fat

12. Chicken with Coconut Sauce

Preparation Time: 15 minutes
Cooking Time: 20 minutes
Serving: 2
Ingredients:

- 1/2 lb. chicken breasts
- 1/3 cup red onion
- 1 tbsp paprika (smoked)
- 2 tsp cornstarch
- 1/2 cup light coconut milk
- 1 tsp extra virgin olive oil
- 2 tbsp fresh cilantro
- 1 (10-oz) can tomatoes and green chilis
- 1/4 cup water

Directions:

1. Cut chicken into little cubes; sprinkle with 1,5 tsp paprika.
2. Heat oil, add chicken and cook 3 to 5 minutes.
3. Remove from skillet, and fry finely-chopped onion 5 minutes.
4. Return chicken to pan. Add tomatoes,1,5 tsp paprika, and water. Bring to a boil, and then simmer 4 minutes.

5. Mix cornstarch and coconut milk; stir into chicken mixture, and cook until it has done.
6. Sprinkle with chopped cilantro.

Nutrition: 200 Calories; 13g Protein; 10g Fat

First Course Recipes

13 . Chicken and Cornmeal Dumplings

Preparation Time: 8 minutes
Cooking Time: 8 hours
Serving: 4
Ingredients:
Chicken and Vegetable Filling

- 2 medium carrots, thinly sliced
- 1 stalk celery, thinly sliced
- 1/3 cup corn kernels
- ½ of a medium onion, thinly sliced
- 2 cloves garlic, minced
- 1 teaspoon snipped fresh rosemary
- ¼ teaspoon ground black pepper
- 2 chicken thighs, skinned
- 1 cup reduced sodium chicken broth
- ½ cup fat-free milk
- 1 tablespoon all-purpose flour

Cornmeal Dumplings
- ¼ cup flour
- ¼ cup cornmeal
- ½ teaspoon baking powder
- 1 egg white
- 1 tablespoon fat-free milk
- 1 tablespoon canola oil

Directions:

1. Mix 1/4 teaspoon pepper, carrots, garlic, celery, rosemary, corn, and onion in a 1 1/2 or 2-quart slow cooker. Place chicken on top. Pour the broth atop mixture in the cooker.
2. Close and cook on low-heat for 7 to 8 hours.
3. If cooking with the low-heat setting, switch to high-heat setting (or if heat setting is not available, continue to cook). Place the chicken onto a cutting board and let to cool slightly. Once cool enough to handle, chop off chicken from bones and get rid of the bones. Chop the chicken and place back into the mixture in cooker. Mix flour and milk in a small bowl until smooth. Stir into the mixture in cooker.
4. Drop the Cornmeal Dumplings dough into 4 mounds atop hot chicken mixture using two spoons. Cover and cook for 20 to 25 minutes more or until a toothpick come out clean when inserted into a dumpling. (Avoid lifting lid when cooking.) Sprinkle each of the serving with coarse pepper if desired.

5. Mix together 1/2 teaspoon baking powder, 1/4 cup flour, a dash of salt and 1/4 cup cornmeal in a medium bowl. Mix 1 tablespoon canola oil, 1 egg white and 1 tablespoon fat-free milk in a small bowl. Pour the egg mixture into the flour mixture. Mix just until moistened.

Nutrition: 369 Calories; 9g Sugar; 47g Carbohydrate

14. Chicken and Pepperoni

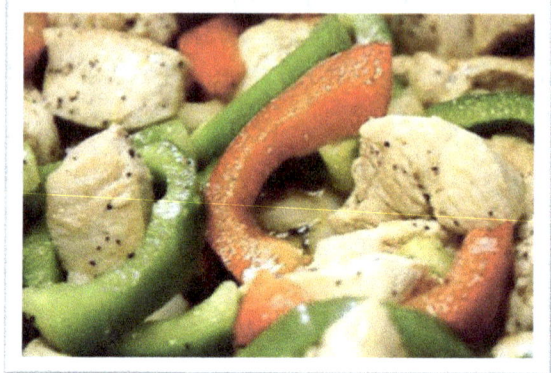

Preparation Time: 4 minutes

Cooking Time: 4 hours

Serving: 5

Ingredients:

- 3½ to 4 pounds meaty chicken pieces
- 1/8 teaspoon salt
- 1/8 teaspoon black pepper
- 2 ounces sliced turkey pepperoni
- ¼ cup sliced pitted ripe olives
- ½ cup reduced-sodium chicken broth
- 1 tablespoon tomato paste
- 1 teaspoon dried Italian seasoning, crushed

- ½ cup shredded part-skim mozzarella cheese (2 ounces)

Directions:

1. Put chicken into a 3 1/2 to 5-qt. slow cooker. Sprinkle pepper and salt on the chicken. Slice pepperoni slices in half. Put olives and pepperoni into the slow cooker. In a small bowl, blend Italian seasoning, tomato paste and chicken broth together. Transfer the mixture into the slow cooker.
2. Cook with a cover for 3-3 1/2 hours on high.
3. Transfer the olives, pepperoni and chicken onto a serving platter with a slotted spoon. Discard the cooking liquid. Sprinkle cheese over the chicken. Use foil to loosely cover and allow to sit for 5 minutes to melt the cheese.

Nutrition: 243 Calories; 1g Carbohydrate; 41g Protein

15. Chicken and Sausage Gumbo

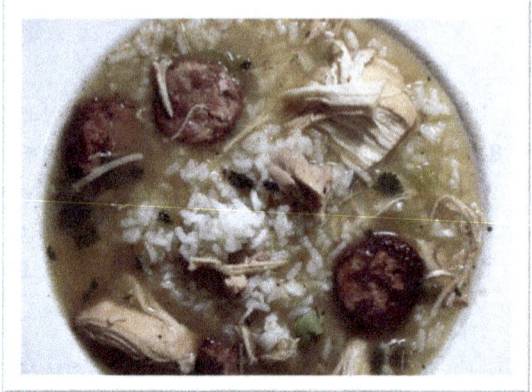

Preparation Time: 6 minutes

Cooking Time: 4 hours

Serving: 5

Ingredients:

- 1/3 cup all-purpose flour
- 1 (14 ounce) can reduced-sodium chicken broth
- 2 cups chicken breast
- 8 ounces smoked turkey sausage links
- 2 cups sliced fresh okra
- 1 cup water
- 1 cup coarsely chopped onion
- 1 cup sweet pepper
- ½ cup sliced celery

- 4 cloves garlic, minced
- 1 teaspoon dried thyme
- ½ teaspoon ground black pepper
- ¼ teaspoon cayenne pepper
- 3 cups hot cooked brown rice

Directions:

1. To make the roux: Cook the flour upon a medium heat in a heavy medium-sized saucepan, stirring periodically, for roughly 6 minutes or until the flour browns. Take off the heat and slightly cool, then slowly stir in the broth. Cook the roux until it bubbles and thickens up.
2. Pour the roux in a 3 1/2- or 4-quart slow cooker, then add in cayenne pepper, black pepper, thyme, garlic, celery, sweet pepper, onion, water, okra, sausage, and chicken.
3. Cook the soup covered on a high setting for 3 - 3 1/2 hours. Take the fat off the top and serve atop hot cooked brown rice.

Nutrition: 230 Calories; 3g Sugar; 19g Protein

16. Chicken, Barley, and Leek Stew

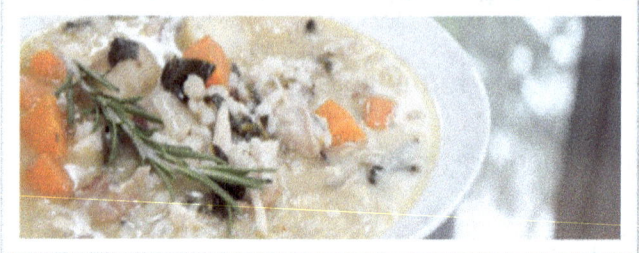

Preparation Time: 10 minutes

Cooking Time: 3 hours

Serving: 2

Ingredients:

- 1-pound chicken thighs
- 1 tablespoon olive oil
- 1 (49 ounce) can reduced-sodium chicken broth
- 1 cup regular barley (not quick-cooking)
- 2 medium leeks, halved lengthwise and sliced
- 2 medium carrots, thinly sliced
- 1½ teaspoons dried basil or Italian seasoning, crushed
- ¼ teaspoon cracked black pepper

Directions:
1. In the big skillet, cook the chicken in hot oil till becoming brown on all sides. In the 4-5-qt. slow cooker, whisk the pepper, dried basil, carrots, leeks, barley, chicken broth and chicken.
2. Keep covered and cooked over high heat setting for 2 – 2.5 hours or till the barley softens. As you wish, drizzle with the parsley or fresh basil prior to serving.

Nutrition: 248 Calories; 6g Fiber; 27g Carbohydrate

Second Course Recipes

17. Sweet and Sour Onions

Preparation Time: 10 minutes
Cooking Time: 11 minutes
Servings: 4
Ingredients:

- 4 large onions, halved
- 2 garlic cloves, crushed
- 3 cups vegetable stock
- 1 ½ tablespoon balsamic vinegar
- ½ teaspoon Dijon mustard
- 1 tablespoon sugar

Directions:

1. Combine onions and garlic in a pan. Fry for 3 minutes, or till softened.
2. Pour stock, vinegar, Dijon mustard, and sugar. Bring to a boil.
3. Reduce heat. Cover and let the combination simmer for 10 minutes.
4. Get rid of from heat. Continue stirring until the liquid is reduced and the onions are brown. Serve.

Nutrition: Calories 203; Total Fat 41.2 g; Saturated Fat 0.8 g; Cholesterol 0 mg; Sodium 861 mg; Total Carbs 29.5 g; Fiber 16.3 g; Sugar 29.3 g; Protein 19.2 g

18. Sautéed Apples and Onions

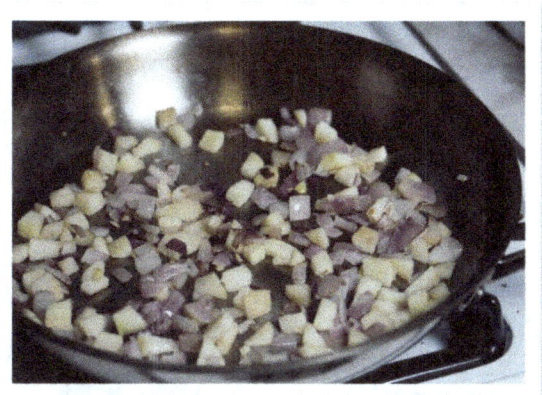

Preparation Time: 14 minutes

Cooking Time: 16 minutes

Servings: 3

Ingredients:

- 2 cups dry cider
- 1 large onion, halved
- 2 cups vegetable stock
- 4 apples, sliced into wedges
- Pinch of salt
- Pinch of pepper

Directions:

1. Combine cider and onion in a saucepan. Bring to a boil until the onions are cooked and liquid almost gone.

2. Pour the stock and the apples. Season with salt and pepper. Stir occasionally. Cook for about 10 minutes or until the apples are tender but not mushy. Serve.

Nutrition: Calories 343; Total Fat 51.2 g; Saturated Fat 0.8 g; Cholesterol 0 mg; Sodium 861 mg; Total Carbs 22.5 g; Fiber 6.3 g; Sugar 2.3 g; Protein 9.2 g

19. Zucchini Noodles with Portabella Mushrooms

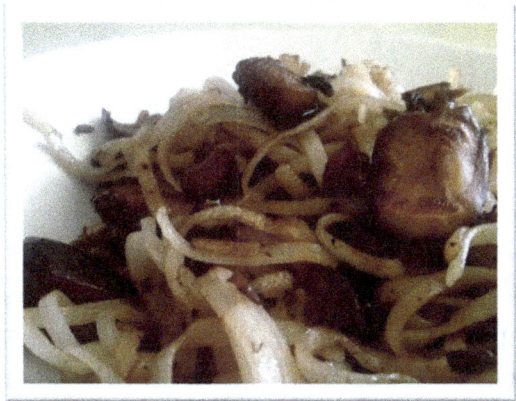

Preparation Time: 14 minutes

Cooking Time: 16 minutes

Servings: 3

Ingredients:

- 1 zucchini, processed into spaghetti-like noodles
- 3 garlic cloves, minced
- 2 white onions, thinly sliced
- 1 thumb-sized ginger, julienned
- 1 lb. chicken thighs
- 1 lb. portabella mushrooms, sliced into thick slivers
- 2 cups chicken stock
- 3 cups water
- Pinch of sea salt, add more if needed

- Pinch of black pepper, add more if needed
- 2 tsp. sesame oil
- 4 Tbsp. coconut oil, divided
- ¼ cup fresh chives, minced, for garnish

Directions:

1. Pour 2 tablespoons of coconut oil into a large saucepan. Fry mushroom slivers in batches for 5 minutes or until seared brown. Set aside. Transfer these to a plate.
2. Sauté the onion, garlic, and ginger for 3 minutes or until tender. Add in chicken thighs, cooked mushrooms, chicken stock, water, salt, and pepper stir mixture well. Bring to a boil.
3. Decrease gradually the heat and allow simmering for 20 minutes or until the chicken is forking tender. Tip in sesame oil.
4. Serve by placing an equal amount of zucchini noodles into bowls. Ladle soup and garnish with chives.

Nutrition: Calories 163; Total Fat 4.2 g; Saturated Fat 0.8 g; Cholesterol 0 mg; Sodium 861 mg; Total Carbs 22.5 g; Fiber 6.3 g; Sugar 2.3 g; Protein 9.2 g

20. Grilled Tempeh with Pineapple

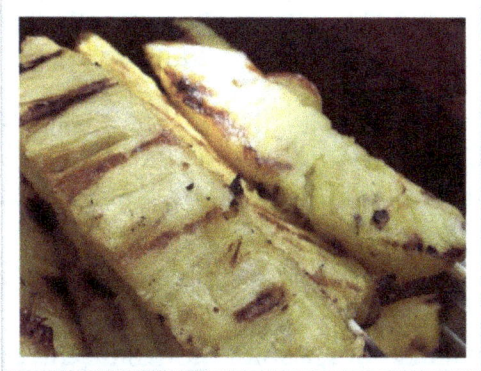

Preparation Time: 12 minutes
Cooking Time: 16 minutes
Servings: 3
Ingredients:

- 10 oz. tempeh, sliced
- 1 red bell pepper, quartered
- 1/4 pineapple, sliced into rings
- 6 oz. green beans
- 1 tbsp. coconut aminos
- 2 1/2 tbsp. orange juice, freshly squeeze
- 1 1/2 tbsp. lemon juice, freshly squeezed
- 1 tbsp. extra virgin olive oil
- 1/4 cup hoisin sauce

Directions:

1. Blend together the olive oil, orange and lemon juices, coconut aminos or soy sauce, and hoisin sauce in a bowl. Add the diced tempeh and set aside.
2. Heat up the grill or place a grill pan over medium high flame. Once hot, lift the marinated tempeh from the bowl with a pair of tongs and transfer them to the grill or pan.
3. Grille for 2 to 3 minutes, or until browned all over.
4. Grill the sliced pineapples alongside the tempeh, then transfer them directly onto the serving platter.
5. Place the grilled tempeh beside the grilled pineapple and cover with aluminum foil to keep warm.
6. Meanwhile, place the green beans and bell peppers in a bowl and add just enough of the marinade to coat.
7. Prepare the grill pan and add the vegetables. Grill until fork tender and slightly charred.
8. Transfer the grilled vegetables to the serving platter and arrange artfully with the tempeh and pineapple. Serve at once.

Nutrition: Calories 163; Total Fat 4.2 g; Saturated Fat 0.8 g; Cholesterol 0 mg; Sodium 861 mg; Total Carbs 22.5 g; Fiber 6.3 g; Sugar 2.3 g; Protein 9.2 g

21. Courgettes In Cider Sauce

Preparation Time: 13 minutes
Cooking Time: 17 minutes
Servings: 3
Ingredients:

- 2 cups baby courgettes
- 3 tablespoons vegetable stock
- 2 tablespoons apple cider vinegar
- 1 tablespoon light brown sugar
- 4 spring onions, finely sliced
- 1-piece fresh gingerroot, grated
- 1 teaspoon corn flour
- 2 teaspoons water

Directions:

1. Bring a pan with salted water to a boil. Add courgettes. Bring to a boil for 5 minutes.
2. Meanwhile, in a pan, combine vegetable stock, apple cider vinegar, brown sugar, onions, gingerroot, lemon juice and rind, and orange juice and rind. Take to a boil. Lower the heat and allow simmering for 3 minutes.
3. Mix the corn flour with water. Stir well. Pour into the sauce. Continue stirring until the sauce thickens.
4. Drain courgettes. Transfer to the serving dish. Spoon over the sauce. Toss to coat courgettes. Serve.

Nutrition: Calories 173; Total Fat 9.2 g; Saturated Fat 0.8 g; Cholesterol 0 mg; Sodium 861 mg; Total Carbs 22.5 g; Fiber 6.3 g; Sugar 2.3 g; Protein 9.2 g

22. Baked Mixed Mushrooms

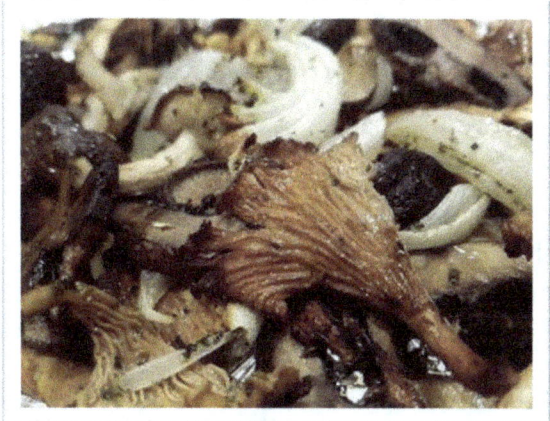

Preparation Time: 8 minutes

Cooking Time: 20 minutes

Servings: 3

Ingredients:

- 2 cups mixed wild mushrooms
- 1 cup chestnut mushrooms
- 2 cups dried porcini
- 2 shallots
- 4 garlic cloves
- 3 cups raw pecans
- ½ bunch fresh thyme
- 1 bunch flat-leaf parsley

- 2 tablespoons olive oil

- 2 fresh bay leaves

- 1 ½ cups stale bread

Directions:

1. Remove skin and finely chop garlic and shallots. Roughly chop the wild mushrooms and chestnut mushrooms. Pick the leaves of the thyme and tear the bread into small pieces. Put inside the pressure cooker.

2. Place the pecans and roughly chop the nuts. Pick the parsley leaves and roughly chop.

3. Place the porcini in a bowl then add 300ml of boiling water. Set aside until needed.

4. Heat oil in the pressure cooker. Add the garlic and shallots. Cook for 3 minutes while stirring occasionally.

5. Drain porcini and reserve the liquid. Add the porcini into the pressure cooker together with the wild mushrooms and chestnut mushrooms. Add the bay leaves and thyme.

6. Position the lid and lock in place. Put to high heat and bring to high pressure. Adjust heat to stabilize. Cook for 10 minutes. Adjust taste if necessary.

7. Transfer the mushroom mixture into a bowl and set aside to cool completely.

8. Once the mushrooms are completely cool, add the bread, pecans, a pinch of black pepper and sea salt, and half of the reserved liquid into the bowl. Mix well. Add more reserved liquid if the mixture seems dry.

9. Add more than half of the parsley into the bowl and stir. Transfer the mixture into a 20cm x 25cm lightly greased baking dish and cover with tin foil.

10. Bake in the oven for 35 minutes. Then, get rid of the foil and cook for another 10 minutes. Once done, sprinkle the remaining parsley on top and serve with bread or crackers. Serve.

<u>Nutrition</u>: Calories 343; Total Fat 4.2 g; Saturated Fat 0.8 g; Cholesterol 0 mg; Sodium 861 mg; Total Carbs 22.5 g; Fiber 6.3 g; Sugar 2.3 g; Protein 9.2 g

Side Dish Recipes

23. Parsley Tabbouleh

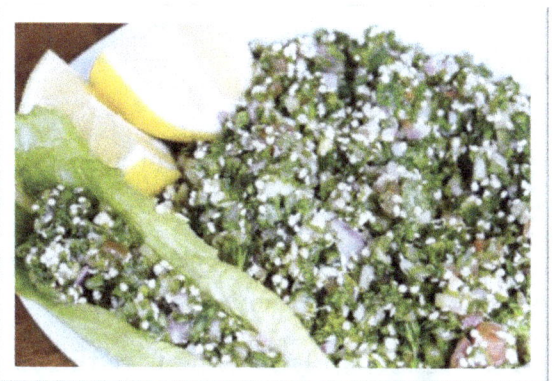

Preparation Time: 5 minutes

Cooking Time: 25 minutes

Servings: 6

Ingredients:
- 1 cup water
- 1/2 cup bulgur
- ¼ cup fresh lemon juice
- 2 tablespoons olive oil
- 2 cloves minced garlic
- Salt and pepper
- 2 cups fresh chopped parsley

- 2 medium tomatoes, died
- 1 small cucumber, diced
- ¼ cup fresh chopped mint

Directions:
1. Bring the water and bulgur to a boil in a small saucepan then remove from heat.
2. Cover and let stand until the water are fully absorbed, about 25 minutes.
3. Meanwhile, whisk together the lemon juice, olive oil, garlic, salt, and pepper in a medium bowl.
4. Toss in the cooked bulgur along with the parsley, tomatoes, cucumber, and mint.
5. Season with salt and pepper to taste and serve.

Nutrition: Calories 110; Total Fat 5.3g; Saturated Fat 0.9g; Total Carbs 14.4g; Net Carbs 10.5g; Protein 3g; Sugar 2.4g; Fiber 3.9g; Sodium 21mg

24. Garlic Sautéed Spinach

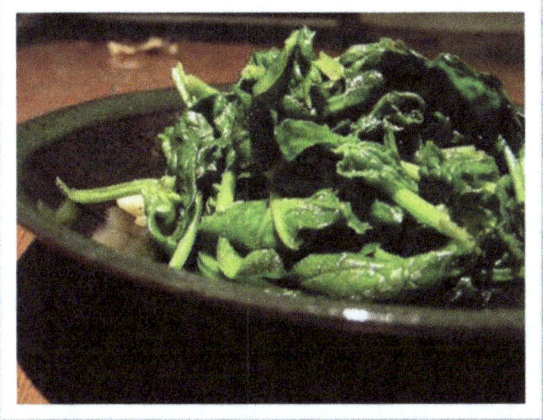

Preparation Time: 5 minutes

Cooking Time: 10 minutes

Servings: 4

Ingredients:

- 1 1/2 tablespoons olive oil
- 4 cloves minced garlic
- 6 cups fresh baby spinach
- Salt and pepper

Directions:

1. Heat the oil in a large skillet over medium-high heat.
2. Add the garlic and cook for 1 minute.
3. Stir in the spinach and season with salt and pepper.
4. Sauté for 1 to 2 minutes until just wilted. Serve hot.

Nutrition: Calories 60; Total Fat 5.5g; Saturated Fat 0.8g; Total Carbs 2.6g; Net Carbs 1.5g; Protein 1.5g; Sugar 0.2g; Fiber 1.1g; Sodium 36mg

25. French Lentils

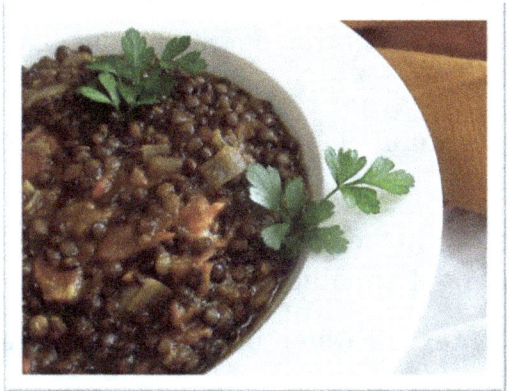

Preparation Time: 5 minutes
Cooking Time: 25 minutes
Servings: 10
Ingredients:

- 2 tablespoons olive oil
- 1 medium onion, diced
- 1 medium carrot, peeled and diced
- 2 cloves minced garlic
- 5 1/2 cups water
- 2 ¼ cups French lentils, rinsed and drained
- 1 teaspoon dried thyme
- 2 small bay leaves
- Salt and pepper

Directions:
1. Heat the oil in a large saucepan over medium heat.
2. Add the onions, carrot, and garlic and sauté for 3 minutes.
3. Stir in the water, lentils, thyme, and bay leaves – season with salt.
4. Bring to a boil then reduce to a simmer and cook until tender, about 20 minutes.
5. Drain any excess water and adjust seasoning to taste. Serve hot.

Nutrition: Calories 185; Total Fat 3.3g; Saturated Fat 0.5g; Total Carbs 27.9; Net Carbs 14.2g; Protein 11.4g; Sugar 1.7g; Fiber 13.7g; Sodium 11mg

26. Grain-Free Berry Cobbler

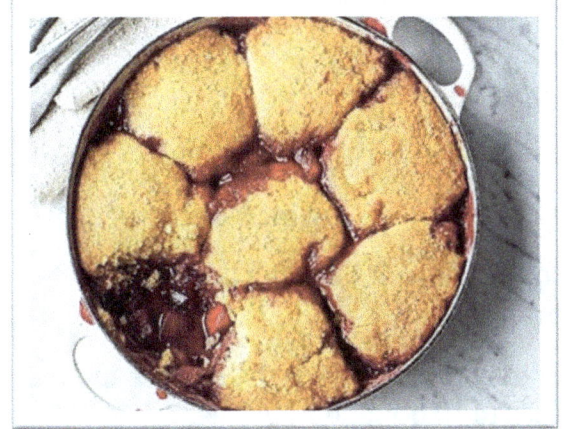

Preparation Time: 5 minutes

Cooking Time: 25 minutes

Servings: 10

Ingredients:

- 4 cups fresh mixed berries
- 1/2 cup ground flaxseed
- ¼ cup almond meal
- ¼ cup unsweetened shredded coconut
- 1/2 tablespoon baking powder
- 1 teaspoon ground cinnamon
- ¼ teaspoon salt
- Powdered stevia, to taste

- 6 tablespoons coconut oil

Directions:
1. Preheat the oven to 375F and lightly grease a 10-inch cast-iron skillet.
2. Spread the berries on the bottom of the skillet.
3. Whisk together the dry ingredients in a mixing bowl.
4. Cut in the coconut oil using a fork to create a crumbled mixture.
5. Spread the crumble over the berries and bake for 25 minutes until hot and bubbling.
6. Cool the cobbler for 5 to 10 minutes before serving.

Nutrition: Calories 215; Total Fat 16.8g; Saturated Fat 10.4g; Total Carbs 13.1g; Net Carbs 6.7g; Protein 3.7g; Sugar 5.3g; Fiber 6.4g; Sodium 61mg

27. Coffee-Steamed Carrots

Preparation Time: 10 minutes
Cooking Time: 3 minutes
Servings: 4
Ingredients:

- 1 cup brewed coffee
- 1 teaspoon light brown sugar
- ½ teaspoon kosher salt
- Freshly ground black pepper
- 1-pound baby carrots
- Chopped fresh parsley
- 1 teaspoon grated lemon zest

Directions:
1. Pour the coffee into the electric pressure cooker. Stir in the brown sugar, salt, and pepper. Add the carrots.
2. Close the pressure cooker. Set to sealing.
3. Cook on high pressure for minutes.
4. Once complete, click Cancel and quick release the pressure.
5. Once the pin drops, open and remove the lid.
6. Using a slotted spoon, portion carrots to a serving bowl. Topped with the parsley and lemon zest, and serve.

Nutrition: 51 Calories; 12g Carbohydrates; 4g Fiber

28. Rosemary Potatoes

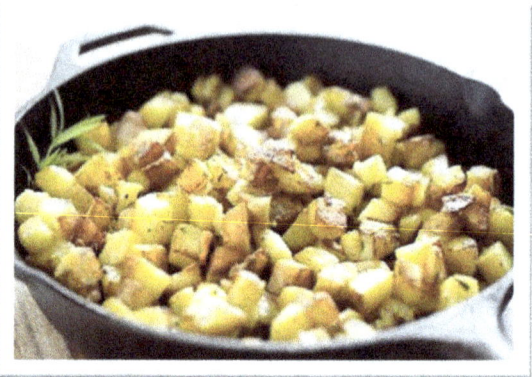

Preparation Time: 5 minutes

Cooking Time: 25 minutes

Servings: 2

Ingredients:

- 1lb red potatoes
- 1 cup vegetable stock
- 2tbsp olive oil
- 2tbsp rosemary sprigs

Directions:

1. Situate potatoes in the steamer basket and add the stock into the Instant Pot.
2. Steam the potatoes in your Instant Pot for 15 minutes.
3. Depressurize and pour away the remaining stock.
4. Set to sauté and add the oil, rosemary, and potatoes.
5. Cook until brown.

Nutrition: Per serving: 195 Calories; 31g Carbohydrates; 1g Fat

29. Corn on the Cob

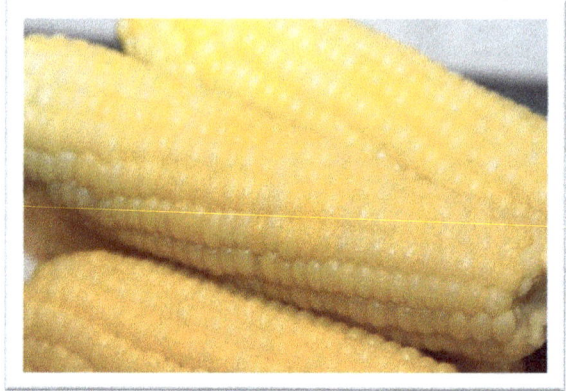

Preparation Time: 10 minutes

Cooking Time: 5 minutes

Servings: 12

Ingredients:

- 6 ears corn

Directions:

1. Take off husks and silk from the corn. Cut or break each ear in half.
2. Pour 1 cup of water into the bottom of the electric pressure cooker. Insert a wire rack or trivet.
3. Place the corn upright on the rack, cut-side down. Seal lid of the pressure cooker.
4. Cook on high pressure for 5 minutes.
5. When its complete, select Cancel and quick release the pressure.
6. When pin drops, unlock and take off lid.

7. Pull out the corn from the pot. Season as desired and serve immediately.

Nutrition: 62 Calories; 14g Carbohydrates; 1g Fiber

Soups & Stews

30. Alkaline Pumpkin Tomato Soup

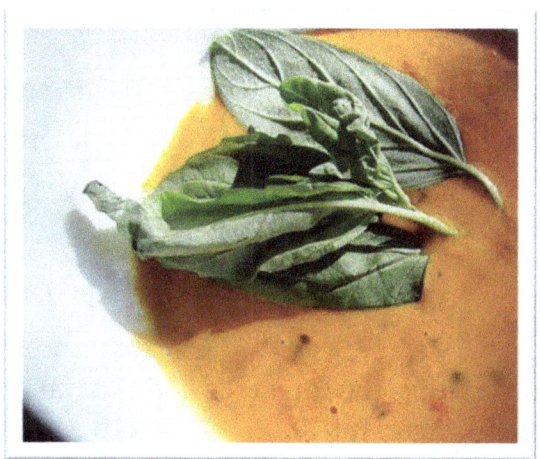

Preparation Time: 15 minutes

Cooking Time: 30 minutes

Servings: 3-4

Ingredients:

- 1 quart of water (if accessible: soluble water)
- 400g new tomatoes, stripped and diced
- 1 medium-sized sweet pumpkin
- 5 yellow onions
- 1 tbsp. Cold squeezed additional virgin olive oil
- 2 tsp. ocean salt or natural salt

- Touch of Cayenne pepper
- Your preferred spices (discretionary)
- Bunch of new parsley

Directions:

1. Cut onions in little pieces and sauté with some oil in a significant pot.
2. Cut the pumpkin down the middle, at that point remove the stem and scoop out the seeds.
3. At long last scoop out the fragile living creature and put it in the pot.
4. Include likewise the tomatoes and the water and cook for around 20 minutes.
5. At that point empty the soup into a food processor and blend well for a couple of moments. Sprinkle with salt pepper and other spices.
6. Fill bowls and trimming with new parsley. Make the most of your alkalizing soup!

Nutrition: Calories: 78; Carbohydrates: 20; Fat: 0.5g; Protein: 1.5g

31. Alkaline Pumpkin Coconut Soup

Preparation Time: 10 minutes
Cooking Time: 15 minutes
Servings: 3-4
Ingredients:
- 2lb pumpkin
- 6 cups water (best: soluble water delivered with a water ionizer)
- 1 cup low fat coconut milk
- 5 ounces potatoes
- 2 major onions
- 3 ounces leek
- 1 bunch of new parsley
- 1 touch of nutmeg
- 1 touch of cayenne pepper
- 1 tsp. ocean salt or natural salt
- 4 tbsp. cold squeezed additional virgin olive oil

Directions:

1. As a matter of first significance: cut the onions, the pumpkin, and the potatoes just as the hole into little pieces.
2. At that point, heat the olive oil in a significant pot and sauté the onions for a couple of moments.
3. At that point include the water and heat up the pumpkin, potatoes and the leek until delicate.
4. Include the coconut milk.
5. Presently utilize a hand blender and puree for around 1 moment. The soup should turn out to be extremely velvety.
6. Season with salt, pepper and nutmeg lastly include the parsley. 7. Appreciate this alkalizing pumpkin soup hot or cold!

Nutrition: Calories: 88; Carbohydrates: 23g; Fat: 2.5 g; Protein: 1.8g

32. Cold Cauliflower-Coconut Soup

Preparation Time: 7 minutes
Cooking Time: 20 minutes
Servings: 3-4
Ingredients:

- 1 pound (450g) new cauliflower
- 1 ¼ cup (300ml) unsweetened coconut milk
- 1 cup water (best: antacid water)
- 2 tbsp. new lime juice
- 1/3 cup cold squeezed additional virgin olive oil
- 1 cup new coriander leaves, slashed
- Spot of salt and cayenne pepper
- 1 bunch of unsweetened coconut chips

Directions:
1. Steam cauliflower for around 10 minutes.
2. At that point, set up the cauliflower with coconut milk and water in a food processor and procedure until extremely smooth.
3. Include new lime squeeze, salt and pepper, a large portion of the cleaved coriander and the oil and blend for an additional couple of moments.
4. Pour in soup bowls and embellishment with coriander and coconut chips. Appreciate!

Nutrition: Calories: 65; Carbohydrates: 11g; Fat: 0.3g; Protein: 1.5g

33. Raw Avocado-Broccoli Soup with Cashew Nuts

Preparation Time: 10 minutes
Cooking Time: 30 minutes
Servings: 1-2
Ingredients:

- ½ cup water (if available: alkaline water)
- ½ avocado
- 1 cup chopped broccoli
- ½ cup cashew nuts
- ½ cup alfalfa sprouts
- 1 clove of garlic
- 1 tbsp. cold pressed extra virgin olive oil
- 1 pinch of sea salt and pepper
- Some parsley to garnish

Directions:

1. Put the cashew nuts in a blender or food processor, include some water and puree for a couple of moments.
2. Include the various fixings (with the exception of the avocado) individually and puree each an ideal opportunity for a couple of moments.

3. Dispense the soup in a container and warm it up to the normal room temperature. Enhance with salt and pepper. In the interim dice the avocado and slash the parsley.

4. Dispense the soup in a container or plate; include the avocado dices and embellishment with parsley.

5. That's it! Enjoy this excellent healthy soup!

Nutrition: Calories: 48; Carbohydrates: 18g; Fat: 3g; Protein: 1.4g

34. White Bean Soup

Preparation Time: 10 minutes
Cooking Time: 40 minutes
Servings: 6
Ingredients:

- 2 cups white beans, rinsed
- ¼ tsp. cayenne pepper
- 1 tsp. dried oregano
- ½ tsp. fresh rosemary, chopped
- 3 cups filtered alkaline water
- 3 cups unsweetened almond milk
- 3 garlic cloves, minced
- 2 celery stalks, diced
- 1 onion, chopped
- 1 tbsp. olive oil
- ½ tsp. sea salt

Directions:
1. Add oil into the instant pot and set the pot on sauté mode.
2. Add carrots, celery, and onion in oil and sauté until softened, about 5 minutes.
3. Add garlic and sauté for a minute.
4. Add beans, seasonings, water, and almond milk and stir to combine.
5. Cover pot with lid and cook on high pressure for 35 minutes.
6. When finished, allow to release pressure naturally then open the lid.
7. Stir well and serve.

Nutrition: Calories 276; Fat 4.8 g; Carbohydrates 44.2 g; Sugar 2.3 g; Protein 16.6 g; Cholesterol 0 mg

Desserts

35. Pumpkin & Banana Ice Cream

Preparation Time: 5 minutes

Cooking Time: 10 minutes

Servings: 4

Ingredients:

- 15 oz. pumpkin puree
- 4 bananas, sliced and frozen
- 1 teaspoon pumpkin pie spice
- Chopped pecans

Directions:

1. Add pumpkin puree, bananas and pumpkin pie spice in a food processor.
2. Pulse until smooth.
3. Chill in the refrigerator.
4. Garnish with pecans.

Nutrition: 71 Calories 18g; Carbohydrate; 1.2g Protein

36. Brulee Oranges

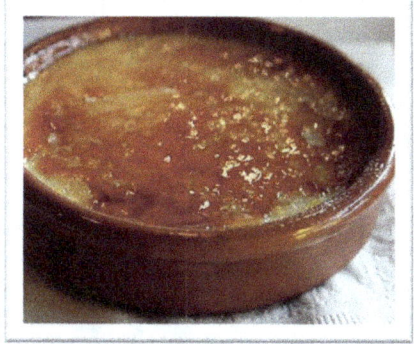

Preparation Time: 5 minutes

Cooking Time: 10 minutes

Servings: 4

Ingredients:

- 4 oranges, sliced into segments
- 1 teaspoon ground cardamom
- 6 teaspoons brown sugar
- 1 cup nonfat Greek yogurt

Directions:

1. Preheat your broiler.
2. Arrange orange slices in a baking pan.
3. In a bowl, mix the cardamom and sugar.
4. Sprinkle mixture on top of the oranges. Broil for 5 minutes.
5. Serve oranges with yogurt.

Nutrition: 168 Calories; 26.9g Carbohydrate; 6.8g Protein

37. Frozen Lemon & Blueberry

Preparation Time: 5 minutes
Cooking Time: 10 minutes
Servings: 4
Ingredients:

- 6 cup fresh blueberries
- 8 sprigs fresh thyme
- ¾ cup light brown sugar
- 1 teaspoon lemon zest
- ¼ cup lemon juice
- 2 cups water

Directions:

1. Add blueberries, thyme and sugar in a pan over medium heat.
2. Cook for 6 to 8 minutes.
3. Transfer mixture to a blender.
4. Remove thyme sprigs.
5. Stir in the remaining ingredients.
6. Pulse until smooth.
7. Strain mixture and freeze for 1 hour.

Nutrition: 78 Calories; 20g Carbohydrate; 3g Protein

38. Peanut Butter Choco Chip Cookies

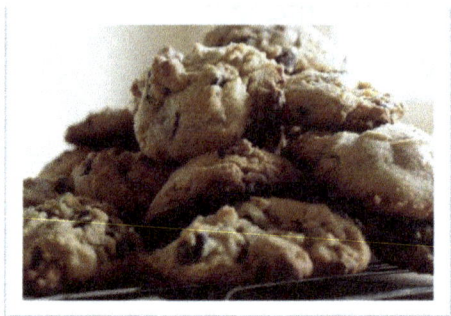

Preparation Time: 5 minutes

Cooking Time: 10 minutes

Servings: 4

Ingredients:

- 1 egg
- ½ cup light brown sugar
- 1 cup natural unsweetened peanut butter
- Pinch salt
- ¼ cup dark chocolate chips

Directions:

1. Preheat your oven to 375 degrees F.
2. Mix egg, sugar, peanut butter, salt and chocolate chips in a bowl.
3. Form into cookies and place in a baking pan.
4. Bake the cookie for 10 minutes.
5. Let cool before serving.

Nutrition: 159 Calories; 12g Carbohydrate; 4.3g Protein

39. Watermelon Sherbet

Preparation Time: 5 minutes

Cooking Time: 3 minutes

Servings: 4

Ingredients:

- 6 cups watermelon, sliced into cubes
- 14 oz. almond milk
- 1 tablespoon honey
- ¼ cup lime juice
- Salt to taste

Directions:

1. Freeze watermelon for 4 hours.
2. Add frozen watermelon and other ingredients in a blender.
3. Blend until smooth.
4. Transfer to a container with seal.
5. Seal and freeze for 4 hours.

Nutrition: 132 Calories; 24.5g Carbohydrate; 3.1g Protein

40. Strawberry & Mango Ice Cream

Preparation Time: 5 minutes

Cooking Time: 10 minutes

Servings: 4

Ingredients:

- 8 oz. strawberries, sliced
- 12 oz. mango, sliced into cubes
- 1 tablespoon lime juice

Directions:

1. Add all ingredients in a food processor.
2. Pulse for 2 minutes.
3. Chill before serving.

Nutrition: 70 Calories; 17.4g Carbohydrate; 1.1g Protein

41. Sparkling Fruit Drink

Preparation Time: 5 minutes

Cooking Time: 10 minutes

Servings: 4

Ingredients:

- 8 oz. unsweetened grape juice
- 8 oz. unsweetened apple juice
- 8 oz. unsweetened orange juice
- 1 qt. homemade ginger ale
- Ice

Directions:

1. Makes 7 servings. Mix first 4 ingredients together in a pitcher. Stir in ice cubes and 9 ounces of the beverage to each glass. Serve immediately.

Nutrition: 60 Calories; 1.1g Protein

42.   Detox Berry Smoothie

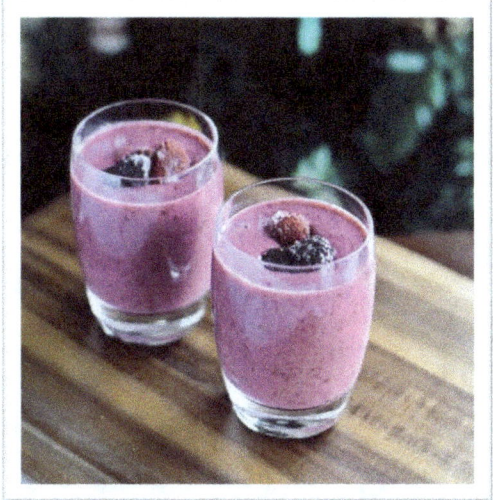

Preparation Time: 15 minutes

Cooking Time: 0

Servings: 1

Ingredients:

- Spring water

- 1/4 avocado, pitted

- One medium burro banana

- One Seville orange

- Two cups of fresh lettuce

- One tablespoon of hemp seeds

- One cup of berries (blueberries or an aggregate of blueberries, strawberries, and raspberries)

Directions:
1. Add the spring water to your blender.
2. Put the fruits and vegies right inside the blender.
3. Blend all Ingredients till smooth.

Nutrition: Calories: 202.4; Fat: 4.5g ; Carbohydrates: 32.9g ; Protein: 13.3g

Other Diabetic Recipes

43. Bruschetta

Preparation Time: 5 minutes
Cooking Time: 10 minutes
Servings: 2
Ingredients:
- 4 slices of Italian bread
- 1 cup chopped tomato tea
- 1 cup grated mozzarella tea
- Olive oil
- Oregano, salt, and pepper
- 4 fresh basil leaves

Directions:
1. Preheat the air fryer. Set the timer of 5 minutes and the temperature to 200oC.
2. Sprinkle the slices of Italian bread with olive oil. Divide the chopped tomatoes and mozzarella between the slices. Season with salt, pepper, and oregano.
3. Put oil in the filling. Place a basil leaf on top of each slice.

4. Put the bruschetta in the basket of the air fryer being careful not to spill the filling. Set the timer of 5 minutes, set the temperature to 180C, and press the power button.

5. Transfer the bruschetta to a plate and serve.

Nutrition: Calories: 434; Fat: 14g; Carbohydrates: 63g; Protein: 11g; Sugar: 8g; Cholesterol: 0mg

44. Cream Buns with Strawberries

Preparation Time: 10 minutes

Cooking Time: 12 minutes

Servings: 6

Ingredients:

- 240g all-purpose flour
- 50g granulated sugar
- 8g baking powder
- 1g of salt
- 85g chopped cold butter
- 84g chopped fresh strawberries
- 120 ml whipping cream
- 2 large eggs
- 10 ml vanilla extract
- 5 ml of water

Directions:

1. Sift flour, sugar, baking powder and salt in a large bowl. Put the butter with the flour with the use of a blender or your hands until the mixture resembles thick crumbs.
2. Mix the strawberries in the flour mixture. Set aside for the mixture to stand. Beat the whipping cream, 1 egg and the vanilla extract in a separate bowl.

3. Put the cream mixture in the flour mixture until they are homogeneous, and then spread the mixture to a thickness of 38 mm.
4. Use a round cookie cutter to cut the buns. Spread the buns with a combination of egg and water. Set aside
5. Preheat the air fryer, set it to 180C.
6. Place baking paper in the preheated inner basket.
7. Place the buns on top of the baking paper and cook for 12 minutes at 180C, until golden brown.

Nutrition: Calories: 150; Fat: 14g; Carbohydrates: 3g; Protein: 11g; Sugar: 8g; Cholesterol: 0mg

45. Blueberry Buns

Preparation Time: 10 minutes

Cooking Time: 12 minutes

Servings: 6

Ingredients:

- 240g all-purpose flour
- 50g granulated sugar
- 8g baking powder
- 2g of salt
- 85g chopped cold butter
- 85g of fresh blueberries
- 3g grated fresh ginger
- 113 ml whipping cream
- 2 large eggs
- 4 ml vanilla extract
- 5 ml of water

Directions:
1. Put sugar, flour, baking powder and salt in a large bowl.
2. Put the butter with the flour using a blender or your hands until the mixture resembles thick crumbs.
3. Mix the blueberries and ginger in the flour mixture and set aside
4. Mix the whipping cream, 1 egg and the vanilla extract in a different container.
5. Put the cream mixture with the flour mixture until combined.
6. Shape the dough until it reaches a thickness of approximately 38 mm and cut it into eighths.
7. Spread the buns with a combination of egg and water. Set aside Preheat the air fryer set it to 180C.
8. Place baking paper in the preheated inner basket and place the buns on top of the paper. Cook for 12 minutes at 180C, until golden brown

Nutrition: Calories: 105; Fat: 1.64g; Carbohydrates: 20.09g; Protein: 2.43g; Sugar: 2.1g; Cholesterol: 0mg

46. Cauliflower Potato Mash

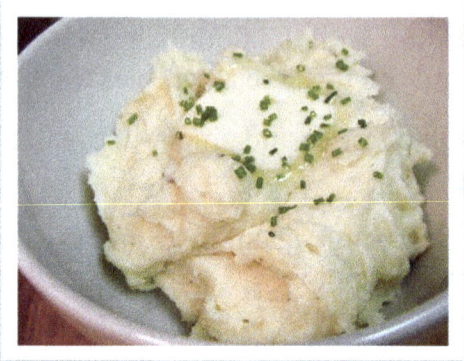

Preparation Time: 30 minutes Servings: 4

Cooking Time: 5 minutes

Ingredients:

- 2 cups potatoes, peeled and cubed
- 2 tbsp. butter
- ¼ cup milk
- 10 oz. cauliflower florets
- ¾ tsp. salt

Directions:

1. Add water to the saucepan and bring to boil.
2. Reduce heat and simmer for 10 minutes.
3. Drain vegetables well. Transfer vegetables, butter, milk, and salt in a blender and blend until smooth.
4. Serve and enjoy.

Nutrition: Calories 128; Fat 6.2 g; Sugar 3.3 g; Protein 3.2 g; Cholesterol 17 mg

47. French toast in Sticks

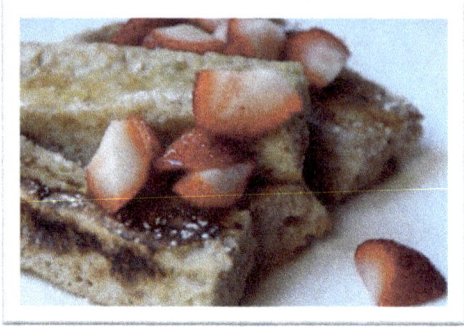

Preparation Time: 5 minutes

Cooking Time: 10 minutes

Servings: 4

Ingredients:

- 4 slices of white bread, 38 mm thick, preferably hard
- 2 eggs
- 60 ml of milk
- 15 ml maple sauce
- 2 ml vanilla extract
- Nonstick Spray Oil
- 38g of sugar
- 3ground cinnamon
- Maple syrup, to serve
- Sugar to sprinkle

Directions:

1. Cut each slice of bread into thirds making 12 pieces. Place sideways
2. Beat the eggs, milk, maple syrup and vanilla.
3. Preheat the air fryer, set it to 175C.
4. Dip the sliced bread in the egg mixture and place it in the preheated air fryer. Sprinkle French toast generously with oil spray.
5. Cook French toast for 10 minutes at 175C. Turn the toast halfway through cooking.
6. Mix the sugar and cinnamon in a bowl.
7. Cover the French toast with the sugar and cinnamon mixture when you have finished cooking.
8. Serve with Maple syrup and sprinkle with powdered sugar

Nutrition: Calories 128; Fat 6.2 g; Carbohydrates 16.3 g; Sugar 3.3 g; Protein 3.2 g; Cholesterol 17 mg

48. Muffins Sandwich

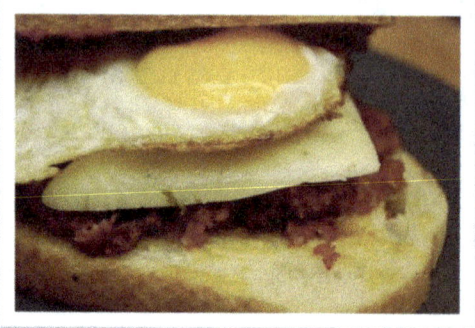

Preparation Time: 2 minutes
Cooking Time: 10 minutes
Servings: 1
Ingredients:
- Nonstick Spray Oil
- 1 slice of white cheddar cheese
- 1 slice of Canadian bacon
- 1 English muffin, divided
- 15 ml hot water
- 1 large egg
- Salt and pepper to taste

Directions:
1. Spray the inside of an 85g mold with oil spray and place it in the air fryer.
2. Preheat the air fryer, set it to 160C.

3. Add the Canadian cheese and bacon in the preheated air fryer.
4. Pour the hot water and the egg into the hot pan and season with salt and pepper.
5. Select Bread, set to 10 minutes.
6. Take out the English muffins after 7 minutes, leaving the egg for the full time.
7. Build your sandwich by placing the cooked egg on top of the English muffing and serve

Nutrition: Calories 400; Fat 26g; Carbohydrates 26g; Sugar 15 g; Protein 3 g; Cholesterol 155 mg

49. Bacon BBQ

Preparation Time: 2 minutes

Cooking Time: 8 minutes

Servings: 2

Ingredients:

- 13g dark brown sugar
- 5g chili powder
- 1g ground cumin
- 1g cayenne pepper
- 4 slices of bacon, cut in half

Directions:

1. Mix seasonings until well combined.
2. Dip the bacon in the dressing until it is completely covered. Leave aside.
3. Preheat the air fryer, set it to 160C.
4. Place the bacon in the preheated air fryer
5. Select Bacon and press Start/Pause.

Nutrition: Calories: 1124; Fat: 72g; Carbohydrates: 59g; Protein: 49g; Sugar: 11g; Cholesterol: 77mg

Conclusion

Diabetes can occur at any age. However, being too young or too old means your body is not in its best form, and therefore, this increases the risk of developing diabetes.

Being diagnosed with diabetes will bring some major changes in your lifestyle. From the time you are diagnosed with it, it would always be a constant battle with food. You need to become a lot more careful with your food choices and the quantity that you ate. Every meal will feel like a major effort. Recent studies show that developing healthy eating habits and following diets that are low in carbs, losing excess weight, and leading an active lifestyle can help to protect you from developing diabetes, especially diabetes type 2, by minimizing the risk factors of developing the disorder.

Too many carbohydrates can lead to insulin sensitivity and pancreatic fatigue, as well as weight gain with all its associated risk factors for cardiovascular disease and hypertension. The solution is to lower your sugar intake, therefore, decrease your body's need for insulin and increase the burning of fat in your body.

When your body is low on sugars, it will be forced to use a subsequent molecule to burn for energy; in that case, this will be fat. The burning of fat will lead you to lose weight.

www.ingramcontent.com/pod-product-compliance
Lightning Source LLC
Chambersburg PA
CBHW070932080526
44589CB00013B/1487